Freedom from Smoke: A Comprehensive Guide to Quitting Smoking

Table of Contents

Introduction

If you are here, I would like to congratulate you on taking the first step towards a smoke-free life!

This is a significant and empowering decision that marks the beginning of a healthier, more vibrant chapter for you. By choosing to quit smoking, you're investing in your well-being and committing to a future filled with greater energy, improved health, and increased longevity.

Your determination to make this change is commendable and will pave the way for numerous positive transformations in your life.

Quitting smoking is indeed a challenging journey, but it's one filled with hope and the promise of a better future. The process of overcoming this habit requires not only a strong commitment but also a resilient mindset. It's about more than just breaking free from nicotine; it's about transforming your lifestyle and embracing new, healthier habits.

Cigarette smoking poses a serious threat to nearly every organ in the body, leading to a wide array of diseases and overall deterioration in health. The harmful effects of smoking are pervasive, as it contributes to chronic conditions such as heart disease, stroke, chronic obstructive pulmonary disease (COPD), and various cancers, including lung cancer.

The toxins in cigarette smoke damage cells, weaken the immune system and impair vital organs, which collectively undermines the body's ability to function optimally. This widespread damage significantly impacts the quality of life and can lead to premature death.

On the other hand, quitting smoking offers profound health benefits and can dramatically improve your quality of life. By giving up cigarettes, you significantly lower your risk of developing smoking-related diseases. Your body begins to repair itself almost immediately after you stop smoking. Your heart rate and blood pressure drop, lung function improves, and the risk of cancer decreases over time.

In addition to that, quitting smoking can extend your lifespan, as it reduces the likelihood of serious health issues and allows you to enjoy more years of good health. Embracing a smoke-free life not only enhances your well-being but also contributes to a longer, healthier, and more vibrant life.

Each year, approximately 40% of current smokers make an effort to quit, but only 4% to 6% achieve long-term success, meaning that roughly 2% of smokers quit for good annually. It's important to note that quitting smoking often requires multiple attempts, and research shows that around half of all smokers eventually manage to quit permanently.

However, since the 1990s, progress in smoking cessation has slowed. This stagnation is attributed to both a lack of increase in the frequency of quit attempts and a plateau in the success rates of these attempts.

One possible explanation for this trend is that the smokers who have successfully quit so far may have been those who found the process easier, while the remaining smokers, who are often more dependent on nicotine, less psychologically stable, or face additional socio-economic challenges, continue to struggle. This means that the more challenging cases remain, requiring more targeted and effective interventions.

It is also notable that two-thirds of individuals who quit on their own relapse within just two days. This highlights the critical importance of focusing smoking cessation efforts on the initial days of quitting, as this period is crucial for overcoming early withdrawal symptoms and establishing new, smoke-free habits. Tailoring support and interventions to address these immediate challenges can significantly improve the chances of long-term success in quitting smoking.

With the right mindset, you approach this challenge with a positive attitude and the belief that you can succeed. Determination is key – it will drive you to persist through the cravings and setbacks that may come your way. Support from friends, family, or professional resources can provide invaluable encouragement and practical advice, making the path smoother and less lonely.

As you progress, you'll experience the numerous benefits of quitting smoking, from improved physical health and increased energy levels to a brighter, more optimistic outlook on life. This journey will not only enhance your well-being but also contribute to a happier and more fulfilling life overall. Remember, every step you take towards quitting is a step towards a healthier you, and each small victory brings you closer to your ultimate goal.

There are a lot of different views when it comes to someone trying to quit. A common misconception among clinicians, smokers, and non-smokers is the belief that "all smokers can quit smoking if they are just motivated enough." This belief echoes similar statements made about alcohol dependence and depression in the early 20th century, where it was assumed that anyone could overcome these issues solely through personal willpower.

We now understand that while some individuals with these conditions are able to recover on their own, many others require professional treatment to make significant progress. This understanding extends to tobacco use as well; overcoming nicotine addiction often necessitates more than just personal motivation.

Another related misconception is the idea that "95% of all smokers who quit do so on their own." In reality, advancements in smoking cessation treatments have significantly changed this dynamic.

Currently, about one-third of smokers who successfully quit do so with the aid of various treatments. This level of treatment utilization surpasses that seen in the management of alcoholism or obesity.

Despite this, some clinicians may doubt the effectiveness of brief advice, but numerous randomized trials have shown that even short, motivational discussions can significantly increase quit rates. While some healthcare professionals may feel they lack the time to provide such advice, it has been shown that a brief, focused intervention of as little as three minutes can be highly effective.

There is also a concern among some clinicians about potentially embarrassing their patients by discussing smoking cessation. However, exit surveys indicate that most smokers actually view doctors who do not address smoking habits as less competent. This underscores the importance of clinicians actively engaging with their patients about smoking, as even minimal intervention can make a substantial difference in a smoker's journey toward quitting.

Assisting smokers in quitting requires addressing two key processes: motivating them to make an attempt to quit and supporting them through the cessation process once they have decided to stop.

At any given time, the readiness of smokers to quit varies significantly. Research shows that approximately 10% of smokers are actively planning to quit within the next month. In contrast, about 30% are considering quitting within the next six months, another 30% have a more vague or indefinite plan to quit at some point in the future, and the remaining 30% have no intention of quitting at all.

Given this distribution, a substantial portion of clinician interventions must focus on motivating smokers who are not yet ready to make an immediate quit attempt.

This involves engaging those who are contemplating quitting in the near or distant future and encouraging them to take actionable steps toward cessation. Clinicians play a crucial role in increasing the readiness of smokers to attempt quitting, by offering support, education, and motivational strategies tailored to each individual's stage of readiness.

Effective intervention can bridge the gap between contemplation and action, making a significant impact on smokers' decisions to embark on their journey toward a smoke-free life.

In this eBook, you will accompany us on a comprehensive journey toward quitting smoking with a wealth of valuable information, practical tips, and effective strategies designed to support and guide you every step of the way.

Quitting smoking is a complex and multifaceted challenge, and our goal is to equip you with the knowledge and tools necessary to overcome it successfully.

You will discover a range of evidence-based techniques to manage cravings, deal with withdrawal symptoms, and address the psychological and emotional aspects of quitting. Our practical tips will help you navigate the daily hurdles of quitting and establish healthier habits that support your smoke-free lifestyle.

We will also explore proven strategies to maintain your motivation and prevent relapse, ensuring that you have a robust plan in place for long-term success.

Whether you are taking your first steps toward a smoke-free life or seeking to strengthen your commitment, this eBook aims to be your trusted companion, offering encouragement and actionable advice tailored to your journey. We are here to support you in breaking free from smoking once and for all, paving the way for a healthier, more fulfilling future.

Chapter 1: Understanding the Addiction

Nicotine addiction is a complicated exchange of biological, psychological, and social factors. Nicotine is primarily found in tobacco products and is responsible for the addictive nature of smoking and vaping. The science behind nicotine addiction involves exploring how nicotine affects the brain, how it creates dependence and the physical and psychological mechanisms that make quitting so difficult for people.

It acts on the brain by mimicking the neurotransmitter acetylcholine. Neurotransmitters are chemicals that transmit signals between nerve cells (neurons), and acetylcholine plays a role in many functions, including muscle movement, cognitive functions, and arousal. Nicotine binds to nicotinic acetylcholine receptors (nAChRs) located throughout the brain, particularly in areas associated with reward, learning, and memory.

Once nicotine binds to these receptors, it triggers the release of dopamine, a neurotransmitter closely linked with pleasure and reward. Dopamine release in the brain's reward pathway creates feelings of pleasure and reinforcement, making the act of smoking or vaping pleasurable.

Over time, the brain adapts to the elevated levels of dopamine, requiring more nicotine to achieve the same pleasurable effects—this process is known as tolerance. This change in brain chemistry leads to addiction because the user becomes dependent on nicotine to maintain normal dopamine levels and avoid withdrawal symptoms.

The brain's dopamine system is one of the key motivations for nicotine addiction. Dopamine is often referred to as the "feel-good" neurotransmitter because it is released during rewarding experiences, such as eating or socializing. When nicotine stimulates the release of dopamine, it reinforces behaviors that lead to repeated use.

Nicotine's effect on dopamine is particularly powerful because it activates the brain's mesolimbic pathway, also known as the reward pathway. This system connects various brain regions, including the ventral tegmental area (VTA) and the nucleus accumbens, which are involved in the experience of pleasure and motivation.

Nicotine's ability to increase dopamine release in this pathway is what makes it so addictive. Over time, the brain adjusts to these repeated surges of dopamine by reducing the sensitivity of the receptors. As a result, smokers or vapers may need to consume more nicotine to achieve the same effects, further fueling the cycle of addiction.

Hence, quitting nicotine is notoriously difficult, and the reason lies in both the physical and psychological aspects of addiction. When nicotine intake stops, dopamine levels plummet, leading to withdrawal symptoms that make it hard to resist the urge to smoke or vape again.

Nicotine replacement therapies (NRT), such as patches, gum, or lozenges, help ease withdrawal by providing small, controlled amounts of nicotine without the harmful chemicals found in cigarettes. These therapies are designed to slowly wean individuals off nicotine while reducing cravings and withdrawal symptoms.

Nicotine addiction is characterized by both physical and psychological dependence. Physical dependence occurs because the body becomes accustomed to functioning with nicotine in the system. When nicotine levels drop, withdrawal symptoms such as irritability, anxiety, difficulty concentrating, and cravings set in. These symptoms are a result of the brain's chemical imbalances caused by the absence of nicotine. The body craves nicotine to restore those chemical levels to their previous, artificially elevated state.

Psychological dependence, on the other hand, involves the habits and routines associated with nicotine use. Smoking or vaping often becomes linked with certain behaviors or emotions, such as stress relief, socializing, or relaxing. These behavioral cues can trigger cravings even after the physical addiction has subsided.

Nicotine addiction is a complex condition involving changes in brain chemistry, the dopamine reward system, and both physical and psychological dependence. The addictive properties of nicotine are largely due to its ability to hijack the brain's natural reward system, making it difficult to quit once a dependence is formed. Understanding the science behind nicotine addiction can help inform more effective treatment strategies, which often combine pharmacological interventions like nicotine replacement therapy with behavioral therapies to address the various aspects of the addiction.

However, breaking the psychological habits tied to nicotine use can be just as challenging. Many people find that social situations, stress, or certain routines trigger a desire to use nicotine, even after quitting. Behavioral therapies, counseling, and support groups are often essential components of successful quitting strategies, helping people recognize and manage the triggers that lead to relapse.

The dangers of smoking extend beyond the smoker. Secondhand smoke, the combination of smoke exhaled by smokers and smoke from the burning cigarette, exposes others to the same harmful chemicals. Non-smokers, especially children and pregnant women, face increased risks of respiratory illnesses, heart disease, and cancer.

Over time, the brain adjusts to the repeated surges of dopamine caused by nicotine, making it harder for the smoker to experience pleasure from everyday activities. This is why many smokers find quitting so difficult; they not only have to deal with the physical withdrawal from nicotine but also have to relearn how to derive satisfaction and relief from other sources. The addiction becomes a cycle that is hard to break without the right support.

That is why understanding the harmful effects of smoking is the first step toward quitting. Many smokers struggle to quit due to the strong addictive nature of nicotine, but it is never too late to stop. Support systems, such as counseling, medication, and nicotine replacement therapies, can aid in the quitting process. Recognizing addiction as a serious health issue is essential for promoting better health and preventing the devastating consequences of smoking.

Recognizing the harmful effects of smoking on your health begins with an honest assessment of both the physical and mental toll it takes on your body. Smoking harms nearly every organ and leads to numerous chronic illnesses, including cardiovascular disease, lung disease, and cancer. However, the gradual nature of these effects can make it difficult to acknowledge the severity of the damage early on. By understanding the early signs of smoking-related health issues and taking action, individuals can begin to overcome the addiction and its detrimental effects.

Smokers often dismiss initial symptoms, such as frequent coughing, shortness of breath, or fatigue, as minor issues. However, these early warning signs are indications that smoking is already impacting the lungs, cardiovascular system, and overall energy levels. Changes in skin appearance, such as premature wrinkles or dull complexion, are another visible effect, showing that the body is being deprived of oxygen and nutrients. These symptoms are signals that smoking is taking a toll on your health, even if serious diseases have not yet developed.

Mental health can also be a key indicator of smoking's impact. Smokers may experience increased stress, anxiety, or mood swings due to nicotine addiction, despite using smoking as a coping mechanism. This psychological dependency reinforces the cycle of smoking, making it harder to quit. Recognizing how smoking affects both the body and mind is the first step in acknowledging the harm it causes.

Once you recognize the effects of smoking, overcoming them requires a multi-faceted approach. The good news is that the body has an incredible capacity to heal, and the harmful effects of smoking can be reversed or mitigated, often starting soon after quitting. To overcome the damage caused by smoking, individuals should focus on taking the first step, which is making the decision to quit smoking and making it a personal goal.

This decision needs emotional and mental strength because quitting smoking can be very challenging, so most people benefit from seeking professional support from doctors, counselors, and smoking cessation programs that offer guidance and tools to manage withdrawal symptoms and cravings. Nicotine replacement therapies (NRTs), such as patches, gum, and lozenges, can also help gradually reduce dependence on nicotine, while prescription medications like varenicline or bupropion assist in managing cravings and improving success rates.

Another approach is trying to adapt healthy habits like exercise, mindfulness, or hobbies that relieve stress. Exercise helps improve lung capacity, boosts circulation, and reduces unnecessary cravings. Eating a balanced diet and staying hydrated will also support your body's recovery from the damage caused by smoking. It is a process with many ups and downs, so it is important to be kind to yourself if you experience a relapse and stay consistent with your quitting efforts, seek support when needed, and recognize that setbacks are part of the journey. Focus on the progress you've made and return to your plan as soon as possible!

Chapter 2: Building the Determination to Quit

Quitting a habit is a long journey that demands more than just intent. It requires a lot of commitment and a structured approach. It is not something that can be done overnight and is a process that has its own complexities.

And this doesn't just hold true for smoking, in fact, every bad habit that becomes a persistent issue takes a lengthy process involving understanding one's motivations, setting clear goals, and solidifying your resolve.

To make it easier to understand, we will break this process into three main parts. The first one involves exploring the right reasons for quitting. At this stage, you ask yourself *why* you want to quit. The second step involves setting achievable goals, and the last one is strengthening your cause. This last step involves using positive affirmations and visualization to build and maintain the determination to quit.

Assessing Your Personal Reasons for Quitting

Understanding why you want to quit is fundamental to building a strong foundation for your resolve. Your personal reasons serve as powerful motivators and can guide you through the challenges that arise.

1. **Impact on your life:**

   Begin by assessing how the habit affects various aspects of your life. This reflection can provide clarity to your cause and commitment. Ask yourself: How does this habit impact my health, relationships, finances, or emotional well-being? For instance, smoking may compromise your lung health and strain your relationships - quitting will help improve these aspects of your life.

2. **Identify the cause:**

   Understanding what triggers your habit of smoking can help you regulate the triggers and devise strategies that may keep the triggers at bay. These triggers may include stress, boredom, or social pressures. For example, if social pressures are a trigger then this can be managed by changing your social circle by surrounding yourself with non-smokers.

3. **Think long-term:**

   Write down your vision of a life without the habit. What positive changes do you anticipate in the longer run by fighting this habit? Envisioning these changes and imagining yourself turning into a better version of yourself can help reinforce your commitment to the cause.

By quitting smoking, your long-term goal may be to have improved health, more stamina, and, as a result, more savings. It is important that the main goals are ingrained into your brain to keep you on track.

4. **Seek Support:**

Seek out reliable individuals in your social circle who will support you in your cause. Reach out to them and let them know of your decision. This could be a close friend or a family member who can help you when it gets tough during the journey.

Additionally, professional help can also be sought for a more structured support system.

Setting SMART Goals

Okay, so now you know why you want to quit, and your mind and body are fully integrated to work towards this cause. The next step is the "HOW". This involves breaking the journey into smaller, more manageable steps so the process does not become overwhelming. Remember, something is better than nothing and consistency is key - this will only happen when we feel like the situation is under our control and not the other way round.

The first step is to start with a clear, long-term goal. This goal is your ultimate aim and should be Specific, Measurable, Achievable, Relevant, and Time-bound (SMART). For instance, the timeline you have in your head by which you need to quit smoking should actually be practical. Thinking that you will entirely quit smoking in two weeks is not achievable and may put undue pressure on you.

Then, once you are clear on your long-term goals, you break them into smaller milestones that you would want to achieve. Smokers can gradually reduce the number of cigarettes they smoke on a weekly basis, and try alternatives like nicotine patches. And in doing so, it is important to celebrate your milestones.

With every small step achieved, you should celebrate and appreciate yourself for your consistency. Your persistent behavior is what will take you till the end of your journey. It is always important to have a plan in place. Setting the goals isn't enough, one should devise an action plan on how to achieve the milestones within a set duration.

This plan should include specific steps, resources, and strategies to address potential setbacks. For example, if your goal is to quit smoking, you need to regulate your habits, triggers, and surroundings.

Lastly, it is important to review your progress from time to time. Setting SMART goals means nothing if you don't assess their effectiveness. It is important to know how well you are doing or if your action plan is working or not.

If you encounter unexpected challenges or if a particular strategy isn't working, reassess and modify your approach. Flexibility and adaptability are crucial in maintaining momentum and achieving success.

Strengthening Your Resolve

During a long journey like this, losing your determination is normal. Positive affirmations and visualization are powerful tools for reinforcing your commitment and maintaining motivation throughout your journey. It is tough, but not impossible.

It is important to remind yourself every day why you're doing this and who you're doing it for. Positive affirmations help shift your mindset and strengthen your commitment. For example, if you're quitting smoking, building a positive affirmation like "I am doing a favor to my body" can be quite motivating for your subconscious mind as it will memorize that quitting smoking can improve your health greatly.

Similarly, envisioning yourself as a person who is clean can create a positive mental image of your success and the benefits that come with it. Spend a few minutes each day visualizing yourself having achieved your goal. Imagine the feelings of accomplishment and the positive changes in your life. Visualization helps keep you focused on your end goal and reinforces your commitment.

As mentioned before, having the right support matters a lot. But you can also be that support for yourself! You have to cultivate a positive mindset by focusing on your strengths and progress rather than dwelling on setbacks and negative feedback from those around you. Remind yourself that overcoming obstacles is part of the process and that persistence is key. There will be many people who will try to break your determination by telling you how it is impossible to quite, but you need to reinforce your new identity as someone who has overcome the habit. For instance, if you're quitting smoking, think of yourself as a "non-smoker" rather than someone "trying to quit." This shift in identity can make your new habits feel more natural and integral to who you are.

Building the determination to quit a habit involves a comprehensive approach that includes deep self-reflection, strategic goal-setting, and mental fortification. Remember, the path to quitting is often non-linear, and setbacks may occur but we need to be persistent.

Chapter 3: Finding the Right Support System

Quitting smoking is a challenging journey that requires more than just willpower—it often involves a strong, reliable support system. Finding the right support system can significantly increase the chances of success, helping individuals stay motivated, manage withdrawal symptoms, and prevent relapse. A tailored support system can take various forms, including family and friends, professional resources, online communities, and support groups. Each plays a unique role in offering emotional, practical, and motivational assistance throughout the quitting process.

Social support plays a crucial role in helping smokers break free from nicotine addiction and maintain long-term success in staying smoke-free. While the physical withdrawal from nicotine can be managed through medication or nicotine replacement therapies, the psychological and emotional challenges of quitting are often where social support becomes invaluable.

Stress is one of the leading causes of smoking relapses. Many smokers use cigarettes as a coping mechanism for stress, anxiety, or negative emotions. When quitting, learning to manage stress in healthier ways is essential. Social support can provide healthy outlets for stress relief, whether it's through engaging in relaxing activities together, exercising, or simply being there to talk.

One of the primary benefits of social support in quitting smoking is the emotional encouragement it provides. Quitting can be stressful, frustrating, and emotionally draining, especially during periods of intense cravings or withdrawal. Having friends, family, or peers who offer encouragement, listen to your struggles, and celebrate your progress can make the process more bearable. They remind you of the reasons you wanted to quit in the first place, reinforcing your commitment and providing a sense of accountability.

In the event of a relapse, having a support system is crucial for getting back on track. Supportive people understand that quitting smoking is a process and helps minimize the feelings of guilt or failure that often accompany a relapse. Instead of being judgmental, they can offer perspective and help you refocus on your quit journey.

Social support can also help boost confidence, which is vital for those who have attempted to quit before and relapsed. People who feel supported are more likely to believe in their ability to quit and stay smoke-free. This confidence is critical, as many smokers face self-doubt during their quit journey, especially if they experience setbacks.

Many smokers associate smoking with social activities, such as breaks at work or gatherings with friends, making the quitting process feel isolating. When trying to quit, people may feel disconnected from social groups, particularly if their friends or coworkers are smokers. This sense of isolation can increase the likelihood of relapse, as individuals may seek comfort in old routines or social circles that reinforce smoking behavior.

Support from non-smoking friends, family, or quit-smoking groups helps reduce this isolation by providing alternative social connections. Joining smoking cessation groups or online communities allows individuals to connect with others going through the same experience. These groups offer not only advice and shared experiences but also the sense that quitting is a shared goal, which can be highly motivating.

Social support also offers practical benefits that can enhance the likelihood of quitting successfully. Friends or family members can help remove smoking triggers, such as avoiding places where smoking is common or providing distractions during moments of cravings. They can also help by reminding you to stick to your quit plan, whether it's attending counseling sessions, using nicotine replacement products, or tracking progress in an app.

Accountability is another key factor. When someone knows they have shared their goal with others, they feel more responsible for achieving it. Whether it's a weekly check-in or ongoing encouragement, having people who care about your progress can help keep you on track.

Social support is a key element in the success of quitting smoking. It provides emotional encouragement, reduces isolation, offers practical help, and promotes accountability. Whether from friends, family, coworkers, or support groups, social connections make the journey of quitting smoking more manageable and sustainable. By surrounding yourself with supportive individuals, the chances of achieving long-term success in becoming smoke-free significantly increase.

Many smokers use cigarettes as a way to manage their emotions, whether it's to calm nerves, relieve stress, or alleviate feelings of sadness or loneliness. Smoking can become a crutch for dealing with these emotions, which makes quitting difficult without addressing the root cause. Counseling helps uncover these emotional triggers, allowing individuals to recognize why they turn to cigarettes in times of distress.

Engaging in counseling or therapy can be an essential step in addressing the underlying emotional and psychological issues that often contribute to smoking addiction. While the physical dependence on nicotine is challenging, many people smoke to cope with stress, anxiety, depression, or other unresolved emotional issues. Therapy helps identify these triggers and equips individuals with healthier coping mechanisms to prevent relapse.

Therapists can work with individuals to explore patterns of behavior and thought that lead to smoking, offering strategies to manage stress or negative emotions without relying on cigarettes. For instance, cognitive-behavioral therapy (CBT) helps individuals change negative thought patterns and develop healthier responses to stress, reducing the reliance on smoking as a coping mechanism.

Quitting smoking requires learning new ways to cope with the challenges of life without turning to nicotine. Therapy can teach individuals a variety of techniques, such as mindfulness, relaxation exercises, or stress management, that provide relief from cravings and emotional discomfort. By developing these skills, people can face difficult situations without feeling the need to smoke.

In addition, therapy can help individuals set realistic goals for quitting, prepare for potential setbacks, and build resilience. Having these strategies in place makes it easier to navigate the quit journey and stay smoke-free in the long term.

The ritual of lighting a cigarette, the social aspect of smoking breaks, or even the habitual use of cigarettes during certain times of the day (e.g., after meals, or while driving) can create a strong psychological dependence.

Therapy helps break these habits by focusing on behavior modification. Therapists work with individuals to identify the habits tied to smoking and develop new, healthier routines that replace the role cigarettes once played in daily life. This process is crucial in creating lasting change and preventing relapse.

For some individuals, smoking is linked to underlying mental health issues such as depression, anxiety, or trauma. These conditions can intensify the urge to smoke, making it harder to quit. Counseling provides a safe space to address these co-occurring mental health issues, offering tailored interventions that not only support smoking cessation but also improve overall mental health.

Treating these conditions often leads to a higher success rate in quitting smoking, as individuals are better equipped to handle emotional distress without turning to cigarettes as a coping mechanism.

By identifying and addressing underlying issues, therapy helps break the dependence on nicotine, equips individuals with healthy coping strategies, and ultimately supports long-term success in becoming smoke-free.

Chapter 4: Creating a Smoke-Free Environment

Creating a smoke-free environment necessitates a thorough understanding and strategic management of the triggers and cues that prompt smoking. Triggers are events or emotional states, such as stress, boredom, or specific routines, that lead to the urge to smoke.

Cues, on the other hand, are sensory reminders, like the sight of a cigarette pack, the smell of smoke, or even certain social situations, that can spark cravings.

To effectively create a smoke-free environment, one must first identify these personal triggers and cues through self-reflection and tracking smoking patterns.

Once identified, the next step is to address them by altering your surroundings – such as removing smoking-related items and cleaning areas associated with smoking to minimize sensory reminders.

Apart from this, modifying daily routines, such as finding new activities to replace smoking habits and avoiding environments or situations that trigger cravings, is crucial.

Addressing emotional and psychological aspects, like managing stress through healthier methods and seeking professional support if needed, further reinforces a smoke-free environment. By systematically eliminating these triggers and cues and adopting new coping strategies, you can create a more supportive and effective environment for quitting smoking.

Triggers

Identifying triggers for smoking is a crucial first step in creating a smoke-free environment. Start by reflecting on your smoking patterns to understand when and where you typically smoke, paying close attention to the situations, feelings, or activities that prompt you to light up.

To gain a clearer picture, keep a smoking diary for a week or two, meticulously recording each instance of smoking along with details such as the time, location, activity, and your emotional state at that moment. This diary helps in pinpointing patterns and common circumstances that lead to smoking.

Other than that, recognizing emotional triggers is essential, as many individuals smoke to manage stress, boredom, anxiety, or other emotions. By identifying these emotional triggers, you can address the underlying issues that drive you to smoke. Lastly, be aware of environmental cues – specific places, people, or activities that act as reminders or temptations to smoke. This could include locations where you used to smoke, particular social settings, or even times of day when the urge is strongest. Understanding these triggers and cues allows you to proactively manage and modify your environment to support your goal of quitting smoking.

Cues

Eliminating smoking cues is a critical strategy for reinforcing a smoke-free environment and supporting your quit-smoking efforts.

Start by modifying your environment: remove ashtrays, lighters, and any other smoking-related items from your home and car, as these can serve as constant reminders and temptations. Thoroughly clean your living spaces and vehicle to eliminate lingering smoke odors, which can trigger cravings.

Next, change your routine to avoid smoking triggers; if you previously smoked during breaks or while drinking coffee, substitute these moments with new activities such as taking a walk or enjoying a healthy snack.

Establishing these new habits helps break the association between certain activities and smoking. Modify your social interactions by informing friends, family, and colleagues of your intention to quit, so they can support you and help you avoid situations where you might be tempted to smoke.

You can also steer clear of environments where smoking is prevalent or where you have a history of smoking with others. Address emotional triggers by developing alternative coping strategies like exercise, meditation, or engaging in hobbies, and consider seeking professional support from a counselor or support group to manage these triggers effectively.

You can also use visual reminders to keep your motivation high; placing positive affirmations or reminders of your reasons for quitting in prominent locations can reinforce your commitment and help you stay focused on your goal.

Implementing support systems and staying committed are essential components of a successful smoking cessation plan. Start by enlisting help from friends, family, or support groups, as their encouragement and accountability can significantly bolster your efforts to quit. Their support provides motivation, practical advice, and emotional backing during challenging times.

Another important aspect is seeking professional help by exploring smoking cessation programs or consulting with a healthcare provider, who can offer personalized guidance, prescribe medication, or recommend therapy tailored to your needs.

Staying committed involves setting clear, achievable goals for quitting smoking and developing a structured plan to reach them. Celebrate milestones, no matter how small, to maintain motivation and acknowledge your progress. Regularly monitor your progress to identify what strategies are effective and where adjustments may be necessary.

Quitting smoking is a gradual process that requires patience and persistence, so be kind to yourself, embrace setbacks as learning opportunities, and stay focused on your long-term goal of a smoke-free life.

By systematically addressing and eliminating smoking cues and triggers, you can create a more supportive environment for yourself and enhance your chances of successfully quitting smoking.

Smoke-free Zones

Making your home and car smoke-free zones is a vital step in creating an environment that supports your efforts to quit smoking. To start, thoroughly clean both spaces to remove any lingering smoke odors. For your home, this involves washing walls, ceilings, and curtains, as well as cleaning carpets and upholstery.

Use air purifiers or deodorizers specifically designed to neutralize smoke smells and ensure that your living areas are fresh and inviting. Remove any ashtrays present in your car and thoroughly clean the interior. This includes vacuuming seats and carpets, wiping down surfaces, and using odor-neutralizing products to eliminate any traces of smoke.

The next step would be to implement practical changes to reinforce the smoke-free environment. In your home, designate specific areas as smoke-free zones, and clearly communicate these boundaries to all household members. This might also involve removing or hiding any smoking-related items, such as lighters and ashtrays, to reduce temptation.

In your car, avoid smoking in or near it altogether, and maintain it as a smoke-free space by ensuring that no one smokes inside.

You need to adapt your routines to support your smoke-free goals. For instance, if you used to smoke while driving or in particular rooms of your home, find alternative activities to replace these habits, such as listening to music or using relaxation techniques.

Making these changes not only helps to eliminate physical cues associated with smoking but also reinforces your commitment to a smoke-free lifestyle by creating environments that support your decision to quit.

People who are actively quitting smoking have a hard time dealing with social situations and cravings. Here are a few strategies to help you in dealing with them.

Social Situations

Preparing for social situations where smoking might be present is essential for maintaining your commitment to quitting.

Start by planning ahead and anticipating potential challenges at events where smoking could be an issue.

Develop and practice responses for common scenarios where you might be tempted to smoke, so you're ready to handle these situations confidently.

Communicate your decision to quit smoking to friends, family, and colleagues, as their support can significantly help you avoid situations that might trigger cravings; they can assist by choosing smoke-free venues and respecting your smoke-free boundaries.

Opt for social activities and locations that are inherently smoke-free, such as non-smoking restaurants, movie theaters, or sports events, to minimize exposure to smoking triggers.

Prepare polite yet firm responses to offers of cigarettes, such as "No thanks, I've quit smoking," which reinforces your commitment while remaining courteous and immersing yourself in positive, engaging activities that don't revolve around smoking, like hobbies, sports, or social events, to keep your mind and hands busy, thus reducing the likelihood of cravings and reinforcing your smoke-free lifestyle.

Cravings

Managing cravings effectively is a crucial aspect of
maintaining your commitment to quitting smoking. Start by
identifying the specific triggers that lead to cravings, such
as particular times of day, emotional states, or certain
activities, so you can develop targeted strategies to handle
them.

When cravings strike, use distraction techniques to keep
your mind and hands occupied; activities like chewing gum,
drinking water, taking a walk, or engaging in a favorite
hobby can help divert your attention away from the urge to
smoke.

You can practice relaxation techniques such as deep
breathing, meditation, or mindfulness exercises to manage
stress and reduce the intensity of cravings. Staying
physically active is also beneficial, as regular exercise
releases endorphins, which can elevate your mood and
lessen the desire to smoke. If needed, employ nicotine
replacement therapies (NRTs) like patches, gum, or
lozenges, as recommended by your healthcare provider, to
help manage cravings and ease withdrawal symptoms.

Building a strong support network of friends, family, or support groups can provide valuable encouragement and accountability during tough moments.

Set and focus on short-term goals to maintain motivation, and celebrate small victories, such as successfully overcoming a craving or navigating a challenging social situation, to reinforce your commitment and progress.

By preparing for social situations and employing effective strategies to manage cravings, you can maintain your commitment to quitting smoking and build a strong foundation for a smoke-free life.

Chapter 5: Coping with Nicotine Withdrawal

Navigating the initial weeks after quitting tobacco can be quite demanding. During this period, many people encounter nicotine withdrawal symptoms that can be particularly tough to handle. These symptoms often include intense cravings for nicotine, persistent headaches, heightened irritability, and a general sense of feeling down or low.

In the early days, these withdrawal effects may seem overwhelming and may disrupt your daily life. The intensity of these symptoms can vary from person to person, but it's important to remember that this phase is temporary. Over time, the severity of these symptoms will gradually diminish, and you should notice a decrease in their frequency.

As your body adjusts to functioning without nicotine, the discomfort will subside, making it easier to manage daily life. Staying focused on the long-term benefits of quitting and finding effective coping strategies can help ease this transition and support your journey toward a healthier, tobacco-free life.

Managing withdrawal symptoms when quitting tobacco can be challenging, but employing various strategies can help ease the process. One effective approach is to constantly remind yourself of the reasons behind your decision to quit. Reflecting on your motivations such as improving your health, being present for your family, or aligning with your personal or spiritual values can serve as powerful sources of encouragement. These reasons can help sustain you through the toughest moments of withdrawal, providing a strong sense of purpose and resolve.

In addition to staying focused on your motivations, consider using specific coping tools designed to support you through withdrawal. Two such tools are The 4-D's and HALT.

Let's talk about **HALT.**

It is an essential self-care tool and it works by helping you recognize certain signs that can help you in combating a slip or a relapse. HALT stands for Hungry, Angry, Lonely, and Tired. It is a straightforward method involving regularly checking in with yourself to ensure that your basic needs are being adequately addressed. HALT tells you to question things about yourself like: Am I Hungry? Am I Angry? Am I Lonely? Am I Tired?

It is easier to slip into old behaviors when your needs are not being met. This is a perfect way of finding out whether you are having the urge to smoke, or is your body asking for something else.

Am I Hungry?

When you feel a sense of emptiness or a vague craving, it's important to ask yourself if you're actually hungry. This sensation of "something missing" can often lead to confusion about whether you're craving food or nicotine. It's not uncommon to feel like you need "something," but you might not be able to distinguish between a need for nourishment and a desire for tobacco.

Tobacco users sometimes skip meals, opting instead to "smoke a meal" due to the habit of smoking when they're not eating. Now that you've quit smoking, it's crucial not to neglect your meals. Skipping meals or ignoring hunger signals can leave you feeling dissatisfied and increase your temptation to reach for tobacco. Your body needs regular, nutritious food to function optimally, and failing to eat properly can exacerbate cravings for nicotine.

When you're hungry, your addiction might mislead you into thinking that tobacco is the only way to fill that void. To combat this, it's essential to address your hunger by eating balanced, regular meals. By satisfying your hunger with nutritious foods, you help reduce the sense of emptiness and diminish the likelihood of turning to tobacco. Prioritizing good eating habits supports your overall well-being and reinforces your commitment to staying tobacco-free.

Am I Angry?

When you're feeling angry, it's important to evaluate whether you're using that anger as an excuse to smoke. Remember, experiencing anger doesn't diminish your worth or your ability to handle situations effectively. Anger is a natural and valid emotion, but it should not be used as a justification for resorting to tobacco.

It's crucial not to let anger drive you back to smoking. Instead of trying to suppress or escape your feelings with a cigarette, focus on addressing and managing your anger constructively. Using tobacco to cope with anger only compounds the problem and detracts from your progress.

Feeling angry is perfectly normal, but it's how you choose to handle those feelings that matters. To manage your anger effectively, start by acknowledging and confronting it. This self-awareness can help reduce the intensity of your anger and ease the anxiety that comes with it.

Ask yourself, "What am I truly afraid of?" Identifying the root causes of your anger can help you address underlying issues more directly. If you find that your anger is becoming overwhelming or is tempting you to return to smoking, seek support. Reach out to friends, family, or a counselor who can offer guidance and help you stay committed to your goal of quitting. By addressing your anger in healthy ways, you can maintain your progress and continue moving towards a tobacco-free life.

Am I Lonely?

Feeling lonely can be a powerful and challenging emotion, and it can sometimes drive us back to old habits like smoking. It's important to acknowledge that loneliness is a natural emotion and that experiencing it doesn't make you any less valuable or worthy.

However, how you respond to feelings of loneliness is crucial. While it's normal to feel alone from time to time, it's essential to handle these feelings in a way that supports your well-being and aligns with your goals. Using loneliness as a reason to return to smoking is not a healthy or constructive solution.

Instead of succumbing to loneliness, try to cultivate a positive relationship with yourself. Embrace and appreciate who you are, and recognize that your worth isn't diminished by being alone. Developing self-love and self-acceptance can help reduce the impact of loneliness.

There are numerous ways to address loneliness without reverting to smoking. Consider exploring new hobbies or interests that can occupy your time and bring joy. Reach out to a supportive friend or family member to talk through your feelings. Volunteering or getting involved in community activities can also provide a sense of connection and purpose. Seeking counseling or professional help can also offer valuable support and strategies for managing loneliness.

Remember, it takes strength and courage to ask for help and to make positive changes in your life. By addressing loneliness through healthy and constructive means, you can stay focused on your goal of quitting smoking and enhancing your overall well-being.

Am I Tired?

When we're exhausted, we naturally become more vulnerable to cravings and stress. Fatigue can make us feel like our only option for a quick boost of energy is to reach for a cigarette. It's important to recognize that while the urge to smoke may seem like a solution, it's not a healthy or effective way to address your tiredness.

If you find yourself struggling with poor sleep or persistent fatigue, consider incorporating relaxation techniques into your routine. Taking a few minutes each day to practice deep breathing, meditation, or other relaxation methods can help you feel more centered and at ease. People who regularly practice relaxation tend to experience fewer cravings and have a better handle on their overall well-being.

Prioritizing good sleep hygiene is essential. Aim to establish a consistent sleep schedule, create a restful environment, and avoid stimulants before bedtime. Quality rest is crucial for maintaining your energy levels and supporting your overall health.

Remember, taking care of your sleep and relaxation needs is not only important but also a form of self-care. You deserve to feel well-rested and rejuvenated, and managing your tiredness in a healthy way will support your journey to stay tobacco-free.

The 4 D's

As you work towards quitting smoking, you'll likely encounter cravings that come and go. These urges can be particularly intense, especially in the early stages of quitting. Fortunately, cravings typically last only a few minutes, and having effective coping strategies can help you manage these moments more easily.

One practical approach is to use the 4 D's, a set of easy-to-remember techniques designed to help you navigate through cravings and withdrawal symptoms. These strategies can provide you with alternative ways to handle the urge to smoke and support you in staying on track with your quit plan.

Deep Breaths

Deep breathing is a powerful technique to help manage cravings and promote relaxation. To practice deep breathing, start by inhaling slowly and deeply through your nose, filling your lungs completely, as if drawing in fresh air similar to the sensation of smoking, but without the harmful effects. Hold your breath for a few seconds to allow the oxygen to fully enter your bloodstream, then exhale gently through your mouth.

Focus on the sensation of the air leaving your body and release any tension you might be holding. This mindful process helps activate your body's relaxation response, reducing stress and anxiety associated with cravings. By integrating deep breathing into your routine, you can create a sense of calm, diminish the intensity of cravings, and support your overall well-being, making it a valuable tool in your journey to quit smoking and embrace a healthier lifestyle.

Drink Water

Staying well-hydrated throughout the day, especially during moments of craving, is a crucial strategy in your journey to quit smoking. Drinking water not only helps flush toxins out of your system but also plays a vital role in managing cravings. Keeping hydrated can prevent feelings of dryness and discomfort that might otherwise prompt you to reach for a cigarette.

In addition to the health benefits, drinking water can keep your hands and mouth occupied, which can be particularly helpful during a craving. Some people find it beneficial to use a straw when drinking water. This technique mimics the hand-to-mouth motion associated with smoking, providing a satisfying distraction without the harmful effects of tobacco.

By consistently drinking water and considering strategies like using a straw, you can support your body's detoxification process, stay hydrated, and effectively manage cravings, making it easier to stay committed to your goal of quitting smoking.

Distract

When you feel a craving for a cigarette, one effective strategy is to distract yourself by getting up and engaging in various activities. Physical movement can be particularly helpful; consider taking a brisk walk outside to refresh your mind and body. If you prefer to stay indoors, try relocating to a different room or area of your home. For instance, you might grab a carrot stick or a healthy snack and enjoy it in another part of the house.

Engaging in other forms of distraction can also be beneficial. Play some music to lift your spirits, immerse yourself in a book, or flip through a magazine to take your mind off the craving. Social interaction can be another powerful distraction; calling or meeting a friend can provide support and shift your focus away from the urge to smoke.

Many individuals who have successfully quit smoking report that changing their environment or engaging in different activities helps them forget the craving entirely. By keeping yourself occupied and altering your surroundings, you can effectively manage cravings and reinforce your commitment to quitting.

Delay

Many smokers mistakenly believe that cravings for cigarettes last much longer than they actually do, often thinking they persist for 45 minutes or more. However, the reality is that cravings are usually much shorter-lived. On average, a craving typically lasts only about five to ten minutes. By timing your cravings, you can discover the truth and reassess your perception of their duration.

Understanding that cravings are brief can help you manage them more effectively. Even if a craving feels intense, remind yourself that it will likely pass within just ten minutes. To help you get through these moments, utilize the other strategies outlined in the 4 D's. Engaging in activities such as deep breathing, distracting yourself, or drinking water can make the time pass more quickly and reduce the intensity of the craving. By recognizing that cravings are fleeting and employing these techniques, you can better manage your urges and stay on track with your goal of quitting smoking.

Nicotine Replacement Therapy (NRT)

The most extensively researched and commonly used pharmacotherapy for managing nicotine dependence and withdrawal is nicotine replacement therapy (NRT). NRT is available in several forms, including gum, transdermal patches, nasal sprays, oral inhalers, and tablets. Each form offers different methods of nicotine delivery.

The transdermal patch provides a slow, sustained release of nicotine over a period of time, helping to maintain stable nicotine levels throughout the day. In contrast, products like gum, nasal spray, oral inhalers, and tablets deliver nicotine more rapidly, offering immediate relief from cravings and helping to manage acute urges.

These various NRT products differ in their efficacy and the rate at which nicotine is absorbed into the bloodstream. While they are generally more effective when used in conjunction with cessation counseling, they can still be beneficial even without additional behavioral therapy. By providing relief from both general and breakthrough cravings, NRT can significantly support individuals in their efforts to quit smoking. There are several types of NRT products available, each with its own benefits and usage considerations.

Nicotine Patches

Nicotine patches are designed to be applied to the skin, delivering a consistent, steady dose of nicotine throughout the day. These patches come in various dosages, allowing users to select a strength that matches their level of nicotine dependence. For heavy smokers, stronger patches can provide adequate support, while those with lower dependence can opt for lower-dose patches. This flexibility helps users gradually reduce their nicotine intake over several weeks or more, easing their transition to lower nicotine levels and eventually achieving a nicotine-free state.

Evidence supports the safety of long-term use of nicotine patches for maintaining tobacco abstinence. One of the key advantages of nicotine patches compared to other nicotine replacement therapies is their ease of use. Users simply apply a patch in the morning and leave it on for 24 hours, making it a more straightforward option than products that require active use throughout the day. Although nicotine is delivered more slowly with patches than with acute NRT forms, nicotine plasma concentrations can actually peak higher during the day with patches than with other methods.

Nicotine patches are available in various strengths, ranging from 5 mg to 22 mg of nicotine per 24-hour period, which helps to achieve plasma nicotine levels comparable to those seen in heavy smokers. Common side effects include local skin reactions, which can be minimized by rotating the application site daily as recommended. Some users report sleep disturbances with 24-hour patches. Despite these potential side effects, nicotine patches remain a widely used and effective option for supporting smoking cessation.

Nicotine Gum

The first nicotine replacement therapy (NRT) introduced to consumers was transmucosal nicotine polacrilex, commonly known as nicotine gum. Unlike regular chewing gum, nicotine gum is designed to be chewed intermittently and held in the mouth for about 30 minutes as needed to release nicotine. It comes in two dosage strengths: 2 mg and 4 mg. Research indicates that smokers with higher nicotine dependence are more likely to achieve abstinence with the 4 mg gum compared to the 2 mg option. Typically, the number of gum doses per day is gradually reduced over weeks or months until the individual no longer needs it.

To optimize nicotine absorption, users should avoid consuming acidic beverages, such as soda, coffee, or beer, for 15 minutes before and during gum use, as these can interfere with the buccal absorption of nicotine.

Nicotine Lozenges

The nicotine lozenge is available in 2 mg and 4 mg formulations. Unlike nicotine gum, the lozenge is not chewed but instead dissolves slowly in the mouth over about 30 minutes, though this duration can vary among individuals. Nicotine from the lozenge is absorbed gradually through the buccal mucosa and enters systemic circulation.

The lozenge offers an alternative to gum for individuals who prefer not to chew but still need intermittent, controlled nicotine dosing. It generally provides a slightly higher amount of nicotine absorption compared to nicotine gum.

Nicotine Nasal Spray

Nicotine nasal spray is designed to deliver nicotine more quickly compared to other forms of nicotine replacement therapy. The consumer product consists of a multi-dose bottle with a pump mechanism that dispenses 0.5 mg of nicotine per 50 μL spray. Each dose involves two sprays, one in each nostril. This form of NRT is absorbed into the bloodstream more rapidly than other nicotine delivery methods.

Patients typically start with one or two doses per hour, with the possibility of increasing up to a maximum of 40 doses per day. For example, administering one dose of nasal spray per hour (equivalent to 1 mg of nicotine) over 10 hours results in average plasma nicotine concentrations of 8 ng/ml.

Nicotine Inhalers

The nicotine vapor inhaler consists of a mouthpiece and a plastic cartridge filled with nicotine. It was designed to address the behavioral aspects of smoking, such as the hand-to-mouth action, while simultaneously delivering nicotine to help alleviate withdrawal symptoms associated with quitting tobacco. Despite being called an "inhaler," most of the nicotine is actually delivered to the oral cavity (36%) and the esophagus and stomach (36%), with only a small amount reaching the lungs (4%).

The inhaler primarily facilitates nicotine absorption through the oral mucosa, making its absorption rate comparable to that of nicotine gum. Each cartridge contains 10 mg of nicotine, from which up to 4 mg can be delivered, and about 2 mg can be absorbed with frequent use.

Nicotine Mouthspray

Nicotine mouthspray offers a rapid and efficient method for delivering nicotine directly to your mouth, providing a quick solution for managing cravings. The spray is designed to deliver a precise dose of nicotine with each application, allowing for immediate relief from urges to smoke. This form of nicotine replacement therapy is particularly convenient for individuals who need on-the-go support, as it can be easily carried and used discreetly.

The mouthspray works by dispersing nicotine into the oral cavity, where it is rapidly absorbed through the mucous membranes. This quick absorption helps to quickly mitigate withdrawal symptoms and curb cravings, often within minutes of use. Because it is small and portable, the mouthspray can be used anytime and anywhere, making it an accessible option for those who need frequent or immediate nicotine relief.

In addition to its convenience, nicotine mouthspray offers the advantage of being easy to use. A few sprays directly into the mouth can effectively address cravings, making it a practical choice for people who may find other NRT methods less suitable. Overall, nicotine mouthspray provides a fast-acting and user-friendly option for supporting smoking cessation efforts.

Each of these NRT options has its own set of advantages, and the choice depends on your personal preferences and lifestyle. Consulting with a healthcare professional can help you determine the best NRT product for your needs and ensure you use it effectively. They can provide guidance on how to use NRT products, potential side effects, and how to integrate them into your overall quit plan.

Incorporating NRT into your quitting strategy can help ease withdrawal symptoms and improve your chances of achieving a smoke-free life. By exploring and choosing the right NRT option, you can better manage cravings and stay committed to your goal of quitting smoking.

When navigating the challenges of nicotine withdrawal, incorporating alternative coping mechanisms like exercise and relaxation techniques can significantly enhance your ability to manage symptoms and maintain your commitment to quitting smoking.

Exercise

Engaging in regular physical activity is a powerful way to cope with nicotine withdrawal. Exercise helps reduce stress and anxiety, which are common during the quitting process, and can also alleviate some of the physical symptoms of withdrawal, such as restlessness and irritability. Activities like walking, jogging, cycling, or even yoga can boost your mood by releasing endorphins, which are natural mood enhancers. Exercise can help manage weight gain, a concern for many individuals quitting smoking, by boosting metabolism and improving overall fitness. Establishing a consistent exercise routine not only distracts you from cravings but also promotes a healthier lifestyle, reinforcing your commitment to being smoke-free.

Relaxation Techniques

Incorporating relaxation techniques into your daily routine can also help manage withdrawal symptoms and reduce stress. Techniques such as deep breathing exercises, progressive muscle relaxation, and mindfulness meditation can help calm your mind and body. Deep breathing involves taking slow, deep breaths to activate your body's relaxation response, helping to reduce feelings of anxiety and tension. Progressive muscle relaxation involves systematically tensing and then relaxing different muscle groups, which can alleviate physical tension and promote a sense of calm. Mindfulness meditation, on the other hand, encourages you to focus on the present moment without judgment, helping you manage cravings and reduce stress.

Both exercise and relaxation techniques offer valuable tools for managing the discomforts of nicotine withdrawal. By incorporating these strategies into your daily routine, you can improve your overall well-being, enhance your ability to cope with cravings and support your journey toward a healthier, smoke-free life.

Chapter 6: Overcoming Cravings and Temptations

Throughout your journey to quit smoking, you may encounter various reminders of situations where you previously used tobacco, which can trigger a strong desire to smoke again. These triggers can be broadly categorized into several types:

Social Triggers

Being around others who smoke, whether at social gatherings, events, or in casual interactions, can increase your cravings. Social situations where tobacco use was once common or accepted may also prompt the urge to smoke, especially if you're feeling out of place or under pressure to conform.

Emotional Triggers

Your emotions can play a significant role in triggering cravings. Stress, anxiety, boredom, loneliness, sadness, or frustration following an argument can all prompt a desire for tobacco as a coping mechanism. Conversely, positive emotions such as happiness, excitement, or relief can also be triggers, as you might have previously celebrated or relaxed with a cigarette.

Pattern or Activity Triggers

Certain routines or activities that you associate with smoking can serve as powerful reminders. For instance, starting your day with a cigarette, driving in your car, drinking coffee or tea, having a meal, or consuming alcohol were likely tied to your smoking habits. These activities can evoke cravings as they remind you of past smoking routines.

Recognizing these triggers is crucial for developing effective strategies to manage cravings. By identifying what specifically prompts your desire to smoke, you can proactively address these triggers and create new, healthier routines that help reinforce your commitment to quitting.

Successfully quitting smoking often involves managing cravings, which can be challenging but essential for maintaining your commitment to a smoke-free life. Here are some effective strategies to handle cravings and support your cessation efforts:

Understand Your Triggers

Identifying the specific situations, emotions, or routines that trigger your cravings is the first step in managing them. Common triggers include social situations involving smokers, certain emotional states (e.g., stress or celebration), and habitual activities associated with smoking. By recognizing these triggers, you can develop strategies to avoid or cope with them more effectively.

Use Nicotine Replacement Therapy (NRT)

As mentioned in the previous chapter, Nicotine replacement products such as gum, patches, lozenges, nasal sprays, and inhalers can help alleviate cravings by providing a controlled dose of nicotine. These products can reduce withdrawal symptoms and make it easier to resist the urge to smoke. Consult your healthcare provider to find the most suitable NRT option for your needs.

Practice Deep Breathing and Relaxation Techniques

Deep breathing exercises, progressive muscle relaxation, and mindfulness meditation can help manage the stress and anxiety associated with cravings. For instance, taking slow, deep breaths can calm your nervous system and reduce the intensity of cravings. Practicing these techniques regularly can also improve your overall emotional resilience.

Stay Physically Active

Regular exercise can be a powerful tool for managing cravings. Physical activity not only helps distract you from cravings but also boosts your mood and reduces stress. Activities like walking, jogging, or yoga can release endorphins, which can improve your mood and reduce the likelihood of relapse.

Develop Healthy Substitutes

Find alternative activities or habits that can replace smoking. Chewing sugar-free gum, snacking on healthy foods like fruits and vegetables, or drinking water can help satisfy oral fixation and keep your mouth busy. Engaging in hobbies or new interests can also divert your attention away from cravings.

Stay Hydrated and Maintain a Healthy Diet

Drinking plenty of water and eating a balanced diet can help your body recover from nicotine dependence and manage cravings. Staying hydrated helps flush toxins from your system, while a healthy diet supports overall well-being and energy levels.

Seek Support

Reach out to friends, family, or support groups for encouragement and accountability. Sharing your experiences with others who understand the challenges of quitting smoking can provide emotional support and practical advice. Consider professional counseling or therapy if you need additional help navigating cravings and withdrawal.

Plan for High-Risk Situations

Prepare for situations where you anticipate strong cravings. Develop a plan for how you will handle these scenarios, whether it's by using NRT, practicing relaxation techniques, or engaging in a distracting activity. Having a plan in place can help you stay on track and reduce the risk of relapse.

Use Positive Affirmations and Self-Talk

Reinforce your commitment to quitting smoking with positive affirmations and self-talk. Remind yourself of the benefits of being smoke-free and the reasons you decided to quit. Keeping a journal of your progress and celebrating milestones can also help maintain motivation and focus.

By implementing these strategies, you can better manage cravings and increase your chances of successfully quitting smoking. Remember, cravings are a temporary challenge, and with the right tools and support, you can overcome them.

Managing cravings and temptations while quitting smoking can be one of the most challenging aspects of the process. However, effectively distracting yourself during these moments can play a crucial role in maintaining your commitment to a smoke-free life.

Engaging in physical activity is one of the most effective ways to divert your attention from cravings. Exercise not only distracts you but also releases endorphins, which can improve your mood and reduce stress. Activities such as walking, jogging, cycling, or participating in a fitness class can be highly beneficial, and even simple exercises like stretching or a short workout can help manage cravings and keep you occupied.

Pursuing a hobby or interest can also serve as a powerful distraction. Whether it's reading, painting, playing a musical instrument, gardening, or cooking, immersing yourself in a passion or pastime can help take your mind off cravings.

Hobbies provide a sense of accomplishment and joy, which can positively reinforce your journey to quit smoking. Spending time with friends and family can provide support and keep your mind occupied. Engaging in social activities, such as meeting for coffee, attending a social event, or simply chatting with loved ones, can distract you from cravings and offer emotional support. Sharing your experiences with others who understand what you're going through can also provide encouragement and motivation.

Focusing on a project or task can be a useful distraction as well. Whether it's a home improvement project, organizing your space, or working on a personal goal, concentrating on a task can shift your attention away from cravings and provide a sense of satisfaction and progress.

Practicing mindfulness and meditation techniques can help manage cravings by redirecting your focus to the present moment. Techniques such as deep breathing, progressive muscle relaxation, or guided imagery can calm your mind and reduce stress, helping you manage cravings without giving in to them.

Keeping your hands and mouth busy can also help. Using oral substitutes like sugar-free gum, hard candy, or healthy snacks (e.g., carrot sticks or apple slices) can satisfy the oral fixation that often accompanies cravings. Engaging in activities that keep your hands busy, such as knitting, doodling, or playing with a stress ball, can further distract you from the urge to smoke. Implementing a distraction plan by having a list of activities or techniques ready for moments of craving is also beneficial. This might include listening to music, watching a movie, playing a video game, or browsing through a magazine. Having a variety of options allows you to choose what suits your mood and helps keep you engaged.

Creating a "distraction toolkit" with items and strategies for when cravings strike can also be helpful. This might be a box with motivational quotes, a playlist of your favorite songs, a list of fun activities, or a collection of small puzzles or games. Having this toolkit readily available can help you quickly shift your focus away from cravings.

Regularly reviewing your progress and reminding yourself of the benefits of quitting smoking is crucial. Keeping a journal of your journey can help track your achievements and stay motivated. Reflecting on how far you've come and the positive changes you've experienced can strengthen your resolve and help you manage cravings more effectively.

By incorporating these distraction techniques into your daily routine, you can effectively manage cravings and reduce the temptation to smoke. These strategies not only help divert your attention but also support your overall well-being, making the process of quitting smoking more manageable and successful.

Managing Stress

Feeling stressed after quitting smoking is common, as nicotine withdrawal can affect your mood and stress levels. To manage stress, incorporate relaxation techniques such as deep breathing exercises, meditation, or progressive muscle relaxation into your routine. Engaging in regular physical activity, pursuing hobbies, and maintaining social connections can also help reduce stress. Ensure you get adequate rest, as fatigue can heighten stress and cravings. If stress becomes overwhelming, consider seeking support from a counselor or therapist who can provide strategies and tools to help you cope effectively.

By integrating these distraction techniques and stress management strategies into your daily routine, you can more effectively handle cravings and reduce the temptation to smoke. These approaches not only help keep your mind occupied but also support your overall well-being, making the process of quitting smoking more manageable and successful.

Chapter 7: Healthy Habits for a Smoke-Free Life

The lifestyle in which we are raised or that we adopt as we shape our own lives plays a crucial role in our long-term personal development and should be a key consideration in any discussion or analysis of this topic. Historically, smoking has been a significant symbol of a free and modern lifestyle, a trend that persisted through much of the last century. However, the health costs associated with smoking have proven to be severe and undeniable. Despite smoking's somewhat outdated status as a lifestyle choice, it remains a major global public health issue, causing approximately 8 million deaths annually.

Given these statistics, it is vital for society to focus on strategies to prevent smoking initiation, promote cessation, and identify factors that support long-term abstinence from smoking. Quitting smoking is a challenging journey that goes beyond sheer willpower, requiring comprehensive support and tailored strategies. While the decision to quit is a significant achievement, maintaining a smoke-free life can be particularly difficult in social or work settings.

Regular exercise is crucial for managing smoking cravings and alleviating stress, a common trigger for smoking. Whether it's brisk walking, yoga, or gym workouts, physical activity not only reduces cravings but also boosts overall health and mood. Start slowly and build up to avoid injuries, aiming for a consistent routine that provides a healthy distraction and supports your smoke-free lifestyle.

Rather than focusing on restrictive eating, aim to make informed, health-conscious food choices that enhance your well-being and support your quit-smoking efforts. Adopting a nutritious diet is about creating sustainable habits that contribute to a healthier lifestyle and reinforce your commitment to staying smoke-free.

Importance of Nutrition in Smoking Cessation

Adopting a nutritious diet is a crucial aspect of supporting your quit-smoking journey, as it helps ease the transition and promotes overall well-being. When you quit smoking, your body experiences significant changes, and a balanced diet can play a pivotal role in managing these changes effectively.

Nutrition is particularly important in smoking cessation for several reasons. First, it helps manage withdrawal symptoms such as irritability, fatigue, and cravings. A well-balanced diet rich in complex carbohydrates, like whole grains, can stabilize blood sugar levels and reduce mood swings, while fruits and vegetables provide essential vitamins and minerals to support your body's natural detoxification processes.

High-sugar and high-fat foods can lead to feelings of sluggishness, which may tempt you to reach for a cigarette to stay alert. To avoid these pitfalls, focusing on a well-rounded diet can support your journey to a smoke-free life, especially during the challenging period of nicotine withdrawal.

Incorporate a variety of fruits, vegetables, whole grains, and lean proteins into your meals. These foods provide essential nutrients that support overall health and can help manage weight gain—a common concern when quitting smoking. A balanced diet can stabilize your energy levels, reduce irritability, and improve your mood. Hydration also plays a crucial role; drinking plenty of water aids in flushing out toxins and can diminish the urge to smoke.

Many individuals worry about weight gain after quitting smoking, as smoking often suppresses appetite and accelerates metabolism. To address this, adopting a diet high in fiber from fruits, vegetables, and whole grains can help you feel full and satisfied without adding excess calories.

Protein-rich foods like lean meats, beans, and legumes also aid in controlling hunger and maintaining muscle mass. Focus on consuming whole foods and balanced nutrients. Hydration is equally important; drinking plenty of water helps flush out toxins and can diminish cravings. It's also beneficial to avoid excessive caffeine and alcohol, as these can trigger cravings and make it more challenging to stay smoke-free. By incorporating these dietary strategies into your routine, you can enhance your chances of maintaining a smoke-free lifestyle and support your overall health.

Be cautious of trigger foods and beverages, such as caffeine and alcohol, which can exacerbate cravings. For those who find themselves snacking frequently, opt for healthy choices like nuts or fresh fruit. These snacks not only keep your hands and mouth occupied but also help manage blood sugar levels, reducing mood swings and irritability.

Incorporation of Regular Exercise for Physical and Mental Well-Being

We know that staying active is essential for maintaining our physical health, but did you also know that it significantly enhances your overall well-being and quality of life? Engaging in regular physical activity offers numerous benefits that go beyond just keeping your body in shape.

Firstly, physical activity acts as a natural mood lifter. Engaging in regular exercise can alleviate stress, anxiety, depression, and anger. You might be familiar with the euphoric feeling you get after a workout—think of it as a mood booster without any negative side effects. Over time, as physical activity becomes a consistent part of your routine, you'll likely notice a sustained improvement in your mood and overall sense of well-being.

Furthermore, staying active keeps your body fit and capable. Without regular exercise, your strength, stamina, and functionality gradually diminish. As the saying goes, "You don't stop moving because you grow old; you grow old because you stop moving." Regular exercise enhances muscle strength, which in turn supports your ability to engage in other physical activities and maintain overall functionality.

Physical activity also contributes to better health and can help prevent various diseases. Excessive sedentary behavior, such as prolonged sitting, has been linked to increased risks of heart disease and stroke. Studies indicate that adults who spend more than two hours a day watching television may face a higher risk of cardiovascular issues. By staying active, you can lower your blood pressure, boost your good cholesterol levels, improve circulation, manage your weight, and prevent bone loss associated with osteoporosis. These benefits can translate into fewer medical expenses and interventions later in life.

Staying active can help you live longer. While turning 70 might be the new 60, this is only achievable if you're in good health. Regular physical activity can extend your lifespan and improve the quality of those extra years. It helps delay or prevent chronic illnesses and diseases commonly associated with aging, allowing you to maintain a high quality of life and independence for longer.

Regular physical activity offers a host of additional benefits as well. It can assist in quitting smoking and maintaining a tobacco-free lifestyle, boost your energy levels, help manage stress and tension, foster a positive outlook, improve sleep quality, and enhance self-image and self-confidence. Moreover, being active encourages more time spent outdoors, contributing to overall well-being.

The American Heart Association recommends at least 150 minutes of moderate-intensity aerobic activity per week, which can be easily achieved by engaging in just 30 minutes a day, five days a week. Remember, every minute of moderate to vigorous activity counts towards your goal. So, incorporating more movement into your daily routine doesn't require drastic changes—just start with small steps, increase your activity levels gradually, and reduce sedentary time to experience the numerous benefits of a more active lifestyle.

Alternative Therapies

Some individuals explore alternative therapies to assist in quitting smoking. However, it's important to note that there is currently limited evidence supporting the effectiveness of these methods in enhancing your chances of becoming smoke-free. In some instances, these approaches may even lead to increased smoking.

Here are a few alternative methods that people might consider to help stop smoking:

Acupuncture

Acupuncture is a traditional Chinese medicine practice with a history spanning nearly 3,000 years. This technique involves inserting extremely thin needles into specific points on the body to stimulate the immune and central nervous systems and enhance energy flow to targeted areas. Despite the use of needles, acupuncture is generally not painful.

Traditionally, acupuncture is used to address a range of health conditions, including:

- Lower back pain
- Headaches
- Migraines
- Myofascial pain

A 2019 review involving almost 4,000 participants who smoked suggests that acupuncture may aid in smoking cessation. The review found that acupuncture is most effective when used alongside other smoking cessation strategies such as counseling, participation in a smoking cessation program, and moxibustion.

Further support comes from a 2012 literature review, which indicated that individuals receiving acupuncture had significant improvements in smoking cessation rates compared to those who did not receive any treatment. This may be linked to acupuncture's effect on an ear point that corresponds to the vagus nerve, which is involved in transmitting withdrawal symptoms from the parasympathetic nervous system. Stimulating this point may help block these symptoms.

While promising, more research is needed to fully understand the effectiveness of acupuncture for smoking cessation.

Hypnosis

Hypnotherapy for smoking cessation is a therapeutic approach that aims to assist individuals in quitting smoking by targeting their subconscious mind. This method involves guiding the individual into a relaxed, focused state known as hypnosis, where they are more open to suggestions and positive changes. During a hypnotherapy session, a trained hypnotherapist helps the person enter this trance-like state and then provides suggestions designed to alter their subconscious attitudes and behaviors related to smoking.

The process typically begins with the hypnotherapist inducing a state of relaxation, helping the individual become highly focused and open to change. In this state, the therapist offers positive suggestions and affirmations to help reinforce the desire to quit smoking and diminish cravings and habitual behaviors associated with smoking.

Techniques may include visualizing a smoke-free future, associating smoking with negative consequences, and enhancing motivation to quit. After the session, individuals might be given self-hypnosis techniques or affirmations to practice on their own, reinforcing the changes made during the session.

The effectiveness of hypnotherapy for smoking cessation varies among individuals. Some research and anecdotal evidence suggest that hypnotherapy can be an effective tool, especially when combined with other smoking cessation strategies. For example, a review of studies indicated that hypnotherapy might be more effective than no treatment or placebo, though results can be inconsistent. Success rates can differ widely based on factors such as the individual's susceptibility to hypnosis, the skill of the therapist, and the person's commitment to quitting.

Choosing a qualified and experienced hypnotherapist is crucial for those considering this approach. It is important to select a certified professional with a track record in treating smoking cessation to maximize the chances of success.

Hypnotherapy is often most effective when used in conjunction with other smoking cessation methods, such as nicotine replacement therapy (NRT), counseling, or behavioral therapies. Not everyone responds to hypnotherapy in the same way; while some individuals may find it highly beneficial, others may not experience significant changes. Thus, hypnotherapy can be a valuable component of a comprehensive smoking cessation plan, particularly for those who are open to its techniques and actively engage in the process.

Chapter 8: Celebrating Milestones and Staying Motivated

Celebrating Progress

Recognizing and celebrating your progress while quitting smoking is essential for maintaining motivation and reinforcing your commitment to a smoke-free life. Tracking your achievements is a crucial first step. Keeping a detailed record of your progress – whether through a daily or weekly journal, or using a specialized app – provides a clear visual representation of your milestones. Seeing your progress laid out can serve as a tangible reminder of how far you've come and the effort you've invested.

Setting short-term goals can also be highly effective. Breaking your quitting journey into manageable segments, such as the first smoke-free week or month, allows you to celebrate smaller victories along the way. Each milestone achieved brings a sense of accomplishment and makes the larger goal of quitting smoking feel more attainable.

Rewarding yourself for reaching these milestones is another key strategy. Choose meaningful rewards that are unrelated to smoking, such as treating yourself to a movie night, buying a new book, or enjoying a special meal. These rewards not only celebrate your achievements but also reinforce positive behavior and make the process of quitting more enjoyable.

Sharing your successes with friends, family, or support groups can further enhance your celebration. Informing loved ones about your progress and allowing them to share in your achievements provides emotional support and additional encouragement. Their recognition and praise can be highly motivating and affirming.

Reflecting on the positive changes in your health as you progress is also important. Increased energy levels, improved breathing, better taste and smell, and reduced coughing are just a few benefits of quitting smoking. Keeping a list of these health improvements and reviewing it regularly can help reinforce the value of your efforts.

Creating a visual progress chart or calendar can help you track and celebrate your achievements. Marking each smoke-free day, week, or month on the chart provides a visual reminder of your success and a sense of accomplishment.

Acknowledging your ability to overcome challenges and cravings is another way to celebrate your progress. Reflecting on moments where you successfully resisted the urge to smoke can boost your confidence and reinforce your commitment to quitting.

Considering how quitting smoking has contributed to your personal growth is also valuable. Reflect on the skills you've acquired, such as better stress management or healthier lifestyle choices. Acknowledging these positive changes as part of your overall journey can help maintain motivation.

Maintaining a positive attitude throughout your quit-smoking journey is crucial. Focus on the progress you've made rather than any setbacks. Celebrate every victory, no matter how small, and view setbacks as opportunities to learn and grow rather than reasons to give up. Keeping a positive outlook can help sustain your motivation and commitment to a smoke-free life.

Incorporating these strategies into your quitting process can make the journey more manageable and rewarding. Celebrating your progress not only highlights your achievements but also strengthens your resolve to stay smoke-free.

Reward for Milestones

Rewarding yourself for reaching milestones when quitting smoking is a crucial strategy for maintaining motivation and reinforcing positive behavior. Celebrating your achievements helps to make the journey more enjoyable and provides additional encouragement along the way. To effectively reward yourself, begin by choosing non-smoking rewards that promote healthy habits and provide genuine satisfaction. For instance, consider treating yourself to a relaxing massage, purchasing a new book, or enjoying a special outing. The key is to select rewards that are enjoyable and unrelated to smoking, ensuring they serve as positive reinforcement for your efforts.

Setting clear milestones is essential for tracking progress and creating opportunities for celebration. Break down your quit-smoking journey into manageable goals, such as completing your first smoke-free week, or month, or reaching specific targets like reducing cigarette consumption. By setting these milestones, you can more easily recognize and celebrate your achievements, making the process feel more rewarding and achievable.

When choosing rewards, make sure they are personally meaningful and fulfilling. Whether it's a small luxury like a new piece of clothing, a special meal at a favorite restaurant, or an activity you've been looking forward to, the reward should feel significant and motivating. Planning your rewards in advance and associating them with specific milestones can create additional incentives to stay focused and committed.

A reward schedule can help maintain motivation by providing a structured plan for when and how you will celebrate your progress. For example, you might decide to treat yourself after each smoke-free week or month. This structure not only keeps you motivated but also reinforces the importance of reaching each milestone.

Sharing your successes with friends or family can enhance the sense of accomplishment and provide extra encouragement. Celebrating with others, whether through a small gathering or by sharing your progress on social media, can make the celebration more meaningful and provide additional support.

Make sure that the rewards align with your interests and preferences to ensure they are genuinely motivating. Personalizing rewards to fit your likes and hobbies makes them more enjoyable and effective. For instance, if you enjoy art, a reward might be attending a painting class or visiting an art exhibit.

Reflecting on your success is also important. Take time to acknowledge and appreciate the progress you've made and the effort it took to achieve each milestone. This reflection reinforces your success and helps maintain motivation throughout your quit-smoking journey.

Consider choosing rewards that support your overall well-being and complement your smoke-free lifestyle. For example, a new pair of running shoes can encourage continued physical activity, or a cooking class can promote a healthier diet.

Try to be flexible with your reward system. If you encounter setbacks or need to adjust your milestones, don't be discouraged. Adapt your rewards as needed to keep moving forward and stay committed to your smoke-free goals. By incorporating these strategies into your quit-smoking plan, you can effectively celebrate your progress and reinforce positive behavior for the long term.

Relapses

After quitting smoking, the ultimate goal is to maintain your smoke-free status. Even if it has been a significant amount of time since your last cigarette, unexpected cravings can still arise. These cravings might catch you off guard and challenge your resolve to stay smoke-free.

Quitting smoking marks a significant positive change in your life. However, it is crucial to understand that even a single puff can potentially trigger a relapse into regular smoking. The risk of returning to old habits remains a concern, so it's essential to stay vigilant and committed to your smoke-free goals.

It's common for individuals to make several attempts before successfully quitting smoking for good. Each attempt brings you closer to success, as every effort provides valuable experience and insight. If you've faced setbacks in the past, consider them as learning opportunities. The lessons you've gained from previous attempts can be instrumental in strengthening your resolve and improving your chances of quitting permanently. The journey to quitting smoking is unique for everyone, and having support can make a significant difference.

If you're preparing to try quitting smoking again, there are several strategies that can enhance your chances of success. A positive mindset is crucial; remind yourself that each attempt strengthens your resolve and increases your chances of quitting for good. Reflect on your past achievements, even if they were brief, and view any relapses as valuable practice rather than failures. Keeping your reasons for quitting at the forefront of your mind will help maintain your motivation.

Learning from past mistakes is also essential. Identify what led to your previous slip-ups and consider how you might handle similar situations better in the future. Assess what strategies worked well before and what challenges you encountered. By understanding the circumstances that contributed to your relapse, you can develop more effective coping mechanisms. Writing down these experiences can provide clarity and aid in refining your approach for the next attempt.

Planning your next quit attempt thoroughly can make a significant difference. Reflect on what strategies were effective previously and what needs adjustment. Develop a concrete action plan that addresses potential triggers and outlines how you will stay on track. Preparation at the outset is key to avoiding relapse and increasing your chances of long-term success.

When implementing your plan, consider practical steps to reduce smoking temptations. Avoid environments where you might be tempted to ask for a cigarette and try to stay away from people who smoke. Keep nicotine replacement therapy (NRT) on hand as an alternative to cigarettes, and explore different smoking cessation medications if necessary. Ensure that you have the right support system in place and make use of it effectively. If cravings strike, force yourself to wait for at least two hours before deciding whether you need a cigarette.

If you do have a cigarette or two, don't abandon your quit attempt. Discard the remaining cigarettes and continue with your quit plan. Relapse does not mean failure; instead, use it as a learning experience. Set a new quit date, whether it's in a week or a month, and commit to it with renewed determination. Each attempt brings you closer to becoming smoke-free and enjoying the numerous benefits of a better lifestyle.

Chapter 9: Supporting Others in Their Quitting Journey

Supporting a loved one through their journey to quit smoking is incredibly valuable and can significantly increase their chances of success. Here are some key ways you can offer meaningful support:

It's important to understand that quitting smoking is a major challenge. Smoking isn't just a bad habit; it's a complex addiction that can make quitting difficult. Cravings don't disappear immediately, and it often takes multiple attempts to quit for good. Each attempt is a step closer to success, and your encouragement can play a crucial role in their journey. Celebrate their commitment to quitting, even if they haven't succeeded yet, and remind them that persistence is key.

Your relationship style can impact your quitting process. Reflect on how you interact with their smoking habits and consider how these dynamics affect both of you. For instance, if you tend to criticize their smoking or avoid the topic altogether, it might be helpful to adopt a more supportive approach. Recognize their progress, avoid judgment when they have setbacks, and consider if you might also benefit from quitting smoking.

Starting a conversation about quitting can be tricky, but it's important to create opportunities for dialogue. If they express any thoughts about quitting, respond positively and offer your support. Share your own experiences if you're a former smoker, highlighting how quitting has improved your life. Express pride in their decision to quit and reassure them that you're ready to support them through the process.

If they haven't yet brought up quitting, you can gently initiate the conversation. Mention recent news or information about smoking, and ask if they've considered quitting. Approach the topic with sensitivity and be ready to listen to their thoughts and feelings without pressure.

Ask open-ended questions to better understand their quitting journey. Inquire about their motivations, triggers, and challenges, and listen attentively to their responses. Your aim should be to provide support and insight rather than offering unsolicited advice or judgment.

Avoid lecturing or nagging, as this can be counterproductive. Instead, focus on positive reinforcement and constructive support. If they slip up and smoke a cigarette, reassure them that setbacks are normal and help them refocus on their quit plan.

Offer practical distractions to help them manage cravings. Engage in activities together that don't involve smoking, such as going to a movie, taking a walk, or trying a new hobby. Suggesting healthy alternatives and planning enjoyable, smoke-free activities can help them cope with cravings.

Recognize and celebrate every milestone, big or small. Acknowledge their achievements, whether it's a day, a week, or a month smoke-free. Small gestures, such as sending a congratulatory card or planning a special outing, can reinforce their commitment and provide motivation.

You should always be prepared for the long haul. Cravings and challenges may persist even after the initial quitting period. Your ongoing support is crucial, so continue celebrating their successes, offering distractions, and being there for them through the ups and downs. Your encouragement and patience can make a significant difference in their journey to becoming smoke-free.

Sharing your successful quitting story can be incredibly impactful and inspiring for others who are on their journey to becoming smoke-free. When people hear about someone who has successfully quit smoking, it provides them with hope and motivation. Your story can serve as a beacon of encouragement, demonstrating that overcoming nicotine addiction is possible. This hope can be especially powerful for those who are struggling with their own quit attempts, making the goal of becoming smoke-free seem more achievable.

Quitting smoking is often portrayed as a straightforward task, but the reality is that it involves significant challenges and struggles. By sharing your story, you help normalize these difficulties and validate the experiences of those who are facing similar obstacles. This can reassure them that their challenges are a common part of the process and that persistence is key to success.

Your personal experience also offers practical advice and strategies that worked for you during your quit journey. Sharing these insights can be incredibly valuable for others who are searching for effective ways to manage cravings, overcome triggers, or stay motivated. Your story can provide them with concrete ideas and strategies that they might not have considered before.

Moreover, sharing your quitting story fosters a sense of community among those who are trying to quit smoking. It creates an environment where people can support one another, share their experiences, and feel less isolated. This sense of camaraderie can be crucial in maintaining motivation and commitment to a smoke-free life.

Your success story can also encourage others to take action and start their own quit journey. Seeing a real-life example of someone who has successfully quit can empower others to take the first step toward quitting smoking. Your story can prompt them to seek help, join support groups, or try new quitting methods.

Reflecting on your own journey by sharing your story helps reinforce your achievements and build resilience. It allows you to acknowledge your strengths and boosts your confidence in maintaining a smoke-free lifestyle. This reflection can further solidify your commitment to staying quiet and inspire you to continue supporting others.

Sharing your quitting story also promotes awareness and education about the realities of smoking cessation. It helps to raise understanding about the challenges and triumphs of quitting smoking, the importance of support systems, and the benefits of a smoke-free life. Your story contributes to a broader awareness of smoking cessation and its impact on health and well-being.

Advocating for smoke-free environments and policies is essential for enhancing public health and fostering healthier communities. To effectively support and promote these initiatives, a structured approach is crucial.

You should have a deep understanding of the benefits associated with smoke-free environments. Research the significant health risks posed by secondhand smoke, including its links to heart disease, stroke, and lung cancer, particularly affecting children and non-smokers. Gather comprehensive data and statistics to support your arguments. Use this information to educate your community about the critical importance of smoke-free spaces. By raising awareness, you can help others grasp the profound impact that eliminating smoking in public areas can have on overall health and well-being.

You can also connect with local health organizations and advocacy groups dedicated to tobacco control. These organizations are often equipped with valuable resources, campaigns, and expertise that can bolster your advocacy efforts. Actively participate in their events, support their initiatives, and collaborate on projects aimed at promoting smoke-free policies. Building relationships with these groups can amplify your voice and enhance the effectiveness of your advocacy work.

You should get involved in city council meetings, public forums, and other community gatherings where public health policies are discussed. Use these platforms to voice your support for smoke-free environments. Prepare a clear and concise presentation or speech to effectively communicate your position and respond to questions or concerns from the audience. Engaging in these discussions helps ensure that the need for smoke-free policies is recognized and considered in decision-making processes.

Building a coalition of like-minded individuals and organizations that support smoke-free environments can also be an amazing initiative. Organize petitions, community events, or awareness campaigns to demonstrate broad public support for smoke-free policies. Encourage community members to reach out to their local representatives and express their support. A united front can significantly influence policy decisions and increase the likelihood of successful implementation.

Utilize social media and digital platforms to spread awareness and advocate for smoke-free policies. Share informative posts, updates, and calls to action through various online channels. Engage with your audience by encouraging them to share their own stories and support for smoke-free environments. Social media can be a powerful tool for mobilizing support and amplifying your message.

When advocating for smoke-free policies, it's important to provide practical solutions and alternatives for smokers. Promote resources for smoking cessation, support groups, and nicotine replacement therapies. Address concerns about the impact of smoke-free policies on smokers by offering support and resources to help them quit. This approach not only strengthens your advocacy but also demonstrates compassion and understanding.

Conclusion

Quitting smoking is undeniably a challenging journey, but it is one of the most rewarding endeavors you can undertake for both yourself and those around you. The process of giving up cigarettes involves confronting and overcoming a powerful addiction, which requires immense willpower, resilience, and support. However, the positive outcomes of quitting extend far beyond the immediate struggle, impacting various aspects of your life and the lives of those you care about.

Remember, you hold within yourself the power to break free from the chains of addiction and forge a future that is smoke-free. The journey to quitting smoking is undoubtedly challenging, but it is also a deeply empowering process that can transform your life in remarkable ways. The strategies and support outlined in this ebook are designed to equip you with the tools and knowledge needed to overcome the many obstacles that may arise as you work toward your goal of living a healthy, smoke-free life.

Every step you take towards quitting is a testament to your resilience and determination. This journey will test your willpower, but it will also reveal your inner strength and ability to face challenges head-on. By embracing this journey, you are not only addressing a physical addiction but also proving to yourself that you can overcome significant hurdles.

The strategies provided in this ebook offer practical, actionable steps to support you throughout your quit-smoking journey. From managing cravings and withdrawal symptoms to finding effective coping mechanisms and building a strong support system, these strategies are designed to guide you through the process with greater ease.

By applying these techniques, you can develop a personalized plan that fits your needs and increases your chances of success. The more you integrate these strategies into your daily life, the better equipped you will be to handle the challenges that come your way.

Support is a crucial element in successfully quitting smoking. This ebook emphasizes the importance of building a network of support, whether it be through friends, family, support groups, or professional resources. Having people who understand your struggles and can offer encouragement, advice, and accountability will significantly bolster your efforts.

Consider reaching out to healthcare professionals or counselors who can provide personalized guidance and support tailored to your specific needs. The combined strength of a supportive network and professional advice will enhance your ability to stay committed to your goal.

By harnessing your inner strength, implementing effective strategies, seeking support, and embracing the journey with a positive outlook, you can overcome the obstacles and achieve the ultimate goal of living a healthy, smoke-free life. Your determination and the resources provided in this ebook are key to unlocking a future free from the grasp of smoking. Embrace this opportunity to transform your life and enjoy the countless benefits of a smoke-free existence.

Recognize and celebrate every milestone you achieve on your journey to quitting smoking, no matter how small they may seem. Each day without smoking, each successful handling of a craving, and each positive change in your health is a victory worth celebrating. Celebrating these achievements not only reinforces your commitment but also boosts your morale and confidence.

It's important to acknowledge your progress and reward yourself in meaningful ways that support your overall well-being. Whether it's treating yourself to something special, taking a moment to reflect on your accomplishments, or simply sharing your success with supportive friends and family, celebrating these milestones can provide motivation and encouragement to continue moving forward.